a morning cup of
yoga ™

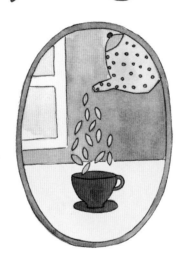

Illustrations by Mary Trechsel Smyer
Pose illustrations by Ernie Eldredge

Published by Crane Hill Publishers
www.cranehill.com

Printed in China

Library of Congress Cataloging-in-Publication Data

Trechsel, Jane Goad.
  A morning cup of yoga / by Jane Goad Trechsel.
    p. cm.
  ISBN 1-57587-172-6
  1. Yoga. I. Title.
  RA781.7 .T74 2002

                          2002008099

10   9   8   7   6   5   4

a morning cup of yoga ™

one 15-minute routine for a lifetime of health & wellness

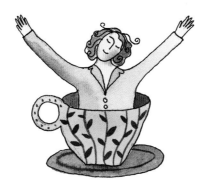

jane goad trechsel

foreword by rodney yee

CRANE HILL
PUBLISHERS

Acknowledgments

I am grateful to the many wonderful yoga teachers I've had along the way, particularly the gifted faculty of the teacher training program at Piedmont Yoga Studio—Rodney Yee, Richard Rosen, Patricia Sullivan, and Mary Paffard.

Thanks to Beth Pierpoint, M.S., P.T., and Garvice Nicholson, M.S., P.T., O.C.S., who reviewed and advised on the exercise routine.

I also want to thank my family and friends who offered support and suggestions; especially my son, Ben, who engineered the CD and my daughter, Mary, whose artwork graces this book.

Contents

Foreword 7

Down the Yoga Path 8

Getting Started 12
    Breathing
    Extra Attention

The Routine...17

If You'd Like to Learn More 61
    Bringing Mind and Body Together
    Improving Your Posture
    Unblocking Your Energy Flow

A Sip of Sutras 64

Meditation..72

An Extra Sip 77

The Routine at a Glance 78

Recommended Reading 80

Foreword

Yoga has taken a new turn in recent years. No longer is it an esoteric practice for an eccentric few. The general public has embraced yoga to utilize its ability to help with general health, stress relief, and overall connectedness. It is helping people deal with their lives and appreciate the abundance of the moment.

People have forgotten how easy it is to start their day with mindfulness, balance, and a swing in their body. With a little yoga to start your day, so many difficulties seem to diminish. Jane shows us the way with a fabulous, easy-to-do yoga routine—*A Morning Cup of Yoga*. The cup is brewed. All you have to do is drink up.

I've known Jane almost ten years, and she always comes through with the highest quality work. Follow along with her as you listen to your body, your breath, and your heart. This is all it takes to wake up on the mindful side of your bed.

Namaste
Rodney Yee

Down the Yoga Path

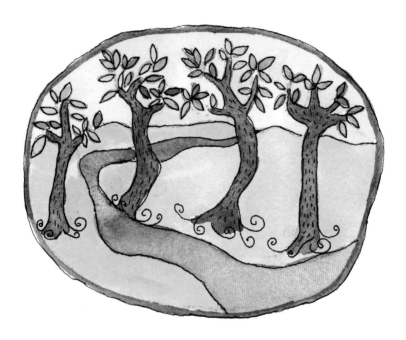

I discovered yoga thirty years ago when I was in my thirties, and it has been my companion and teacher ever since. Yoga's gentle transformation changed me not only physically, but in other ways, too. As time went by, my experience with yoga led me to begin regular meditation, to change my diet, and to generally settle down and become calmer, less judgmental, and less caught up in the little dramas of life. I worked at some of the changes. (Do you know how hard it is to quit smoking?) But some changes I didn't force with willpower. They just happened on their own in a natural unfolding. For instance, I lost my desire for meat. And I didn't give up coffee—it gave me up. I find that on awakening, what I like now is *A Morning Cup of Yoga.*

Here is how this little book began to brew. Many years ago, I made some notes outlining a morning yoga sequence, with a possible title of Yoga in the Kitchen. However, the notes were soon tucked away and sea changes would come about in my life before I pulled them out again. In 1999, I found myself widowed, my children grown with children of their own. I thought, "Well, what do I want to do now?" To sharpen my purpose, I tried an even tougher question: "What would I do if I had only one year to live?"

As luck would have it, yoga master Rodney Yee was offering an advanced studies program beginning in January of 2000 at his studios in Oakland, California. It was to be an intense eighteen-month course—one of the most comprehensive teacher training programs in the country.

Rodney had been one of my yoga teachers for almost ten years. I trusted him and knew the program would be first-rate. I approached him, and he welcomed me to participate. (I considered his encouragement especially kind because I was twice the age of most of the other students who had enrolled.) I said, "My teaching energies may be behind me. If I come, I'm really coming for the fun of it." Rodney laughed and said, "I wish everybody were coming for the fun of it. Come on!"

And so I did. I cleared thirty-eight years' worth of accumulated belongings from my home, enough to rent it out, and drove from Alabama to California, arriving just in time to begin the training. I rented a tiny apartment, sight-unseen, on College Avenue in Berkeley and began a wonderfully vigorous, challenging experience that was both rewarding and fun.

Of course there were some yoga poses that the thirty-year-olds in the class could do easily that I couldn't manage. But I learned to not easily dismiss a pose as unattainable. One can't "attain" a pose anyway. One only approaches it, with awareness, curiosity, and an acknowledgment of whatever restrictions may be present on any given day. This attitude is one of the things that distinguishes yoga from exercise or sport. Yoga changes your mental approach to your body, beautifully uniting body and thought—in ways that many other forms of exercise cannot do.

This was a big lesson. I learned that when the negative voice inside said, "I can't do this!" another, wiser voice could say instead, "This looks difficult. What part of it can I do?" This was a completely different attitude, which freed me to try anything. Perhaps that is why I feel free now to write this book.

People who love yoga want to share it. I've seen students drag reluctant loved ones into class: parents, neighbors, a beloved relative or friend. If they are older, very stiff, or physically restricted in other ways, they often find the first experience to be frustrating. Sometimes they go away discouraged and never try again. And that's unfortunate, because yoga can offer so much to those who need it most. The small routine of stretches and poses in *A Morning Cup of Yoga* can be a gentle entry for any souls who have been thus discouraged or who have not yet tried yoga.

This program can also be beneficial to the serious yoga practitioner. Because it addresses most major muscle groups, it can help to prevent imbalances in the body.

If you have been attending classes, you have already learned that there are many, many poses. Because there is such a rich universe of possibilities, you may choose from among your favorites and avoid those you don't like or can't do. Consequently, it is very possible to end up with an imbalanced program. Because I loved the calming effect of forward bends, I did a lot of them, becoming very flexible. But I wasn't drawn to the strengthening poses, which would have balanced the flexibility. I have some arthritis in a hip now, and I wonder how much of that is age and how much might have been prevented had I adhered to a more balanced regimen through the years.

When I decided to create *A Morning Cup of Yoga*, I wanted a routine that would benefit every part of the body, but would require neither getting down on the floor nor any special clothing or props—a session so brief and accessible that it could become as much a part of daybreak as the morning cup of coffee or tea.

I hope that you will enjoy this routine and will begin feeling the benefits in a very short time. As you begin to feel positive changes in your body and mind, your curiosity may be more and more awakened to the possibilities of yoga. After you have finished your morning routine, you may like to settle down with your breakfast and read the second part of this book. Here you will have a glimpse of the foundations of the yoga system, including a look at the difference between yoga and exercise, the importance of posture, the spiritual precepts of yoga, and how to begin meditation.

And so . . . Good morning! . . . Get ready to stretch . . . Have a sip . . . and enjoy!

Namaste
(The divine in me salutes the divine in you)

Jane Trechsel
Berkeley, California
Spring 2002

Getting Started

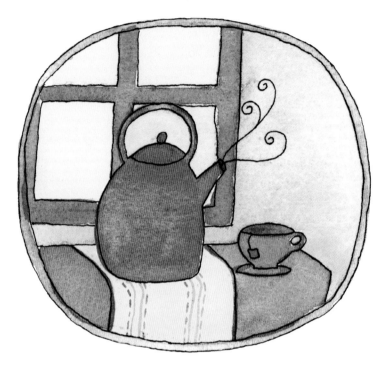

Say hello to your body by incorporating this simple morning routine into your life. You will be amazed at the well-being it produces in even the sleepiest morning body.

Set aside a little more time in the beginning, but once you've learned the routine, you can complete it in about fifteen minutes. Tuck it in while the kettle boils, the oatmeal cooks, in those precious morning minutes alone before your day begins. It is specifically adapted to a kitchen, where you can make use of normal surfaces such as the sink, a counter, a kitchen chair. The routine is all done either standing or sitting, wearing whatever's comfortable, even pj's.

This program is suitable for almost everyone of any age. Even if you are a dedicated fitness buff, you can make this program an invaluable addition to any other practice you have. If you have already lost some strength and flexibility, you will be very pleased at how much you will regain. The body is a living organism, constantly changing and adapting. Nothing about it is fixed or unchangeable. If you have any health problems, however, you should consult your healthcare provider before beginning the program. As you proceed, be gentle with yourself. If you feel dizzy or lightheaded, sit down for a moment and rest.

I have drawn from several yoga traditions to create the Morning Cup program. This gentle, consistent work will give you increased range of motion, more resiliency, flexibility, and strength, and will improve your circulation and digestion. Mysteriously, because of the correlation between movement and other brain functions, yoga is known to yield not only physical, but also emotional and spiritual benefits.

Once you've learned the Morning Cup routine, you can use the sequence I have provided at the end of the book for an easy reference. Or use the CD. It will lead you through the basic routine in exactly fifteen minutes. Cut the sequence out and post it on the refrigerator or bulletin board. (You might want to have it laminated for long-life protection.) Periodically, go back and reread the text to refresh your memory and discover how you may have gotten off track. It's easy to readjust and stay in balance.

Breathing

Conscious breathing is essential as you practice. Attention to breath is one of the crucial offerings of yoga. Our sedentary culture encourages shallow breathing. Think how many hours of the day we spend sitting at desks and computers, or behind the wheel of a car, or in front of the television. When we sit in a slumped position with spine rounded, the chest cavity is compressed, making it almost impossible to fill the lungs with a good breath. Yoga recognizes that the breath is a major pathway for bringing dynamic energy into our bodies. If we deprive ourselves of sufficient air, energy declines, health deteriorates, and our light begins to dim. It's as though we were trying to run a car on a poor grade of fuel.

Remember how Tinker Bell needed the infusion of children's faith to bring back her vitality and make her light shine? We too need infusions . . . of air! Retraining ourselves to breathe deeply can have a wonderfully healing effect. You will be reminded to breathe deeply throughout this program, and I hope that the habit of breath awareness will start to carry into the rest of your day.

In yoga there are many breathing practices, but for the Morning Cup, you'll use just three techniques:

 Ujjayi breath: To get the feel of the *ujjayi* breath, open your mouth and whisper "aaaah" as you breathe in and out slowly. You will notice a slight constriction in your throat, which produces the sound. Now close your mouth, breathe through your nose, and reproduce that sound, both as you inhale and as you exhale. Hearing the breath will help you to monitor it, keeping it slow, smooth, and deep. An added benefit is that the *ujjayi* breath has a strengthening effect on the bronchial system.

Double breathing: Inhalation is broken into two segments; the first one is a short sniff, the second a longer, deeper inhalation. The exhale is also two-part; exhale through your open mouth twice, saying in a loud whisper, "Ha-haaaaaaah." I have indicated the poses within the routine where this breath would be suitable. Double breathing brings breath deep into the lungs and works particularly well with the dynamic, or actively moving, parts of the routine.

Silent breath: Breathe deeply, slowly, and rhythmically, but very quietly.

Throughout the Morning Cup program, I will suggest using one of these three breaths. All of these techniques will improve your lung strength, oxygenate the cells of the body, and help your light to shine brighter.

Extra Attention

I have added an "Extra Attention" box for some of the movements. These notes may guide you to expand your awareness and explore your experience at more subtle levels, thus deepening your relationship with your body. In the beginning, just focus on the basic instructions. Then, as you become familiar with the work, the "Extra Attention" boxes will be more meaningful.

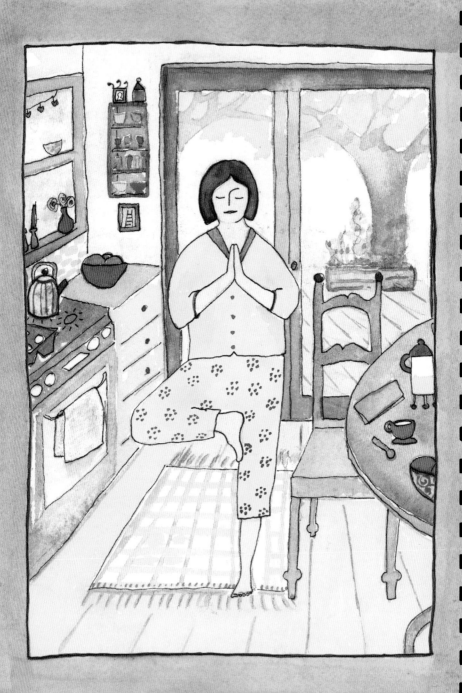

The Routine

Simple morning stretches to enjoy every day

The basic program can be done in fifteen minutes. The CD in the back of the book will lead you through the routine in exactly that time. However, please read the book carefully, and get familiar with the work before using the CD. On mornings when you have more leisure, you can linger in the poses, increase repetitions, and try some of the optional work. The sequence is designed to warm up and stretch different parts of your body in a balanced way, so don't skip around.

Before you begin this or any exercise program consult your healthcare provider. If a movement causes discomfort, skip it.

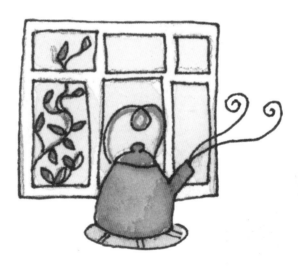

Warm-up 1

Breath: double breathing

1. Stand with feet a comfortable distance apart.

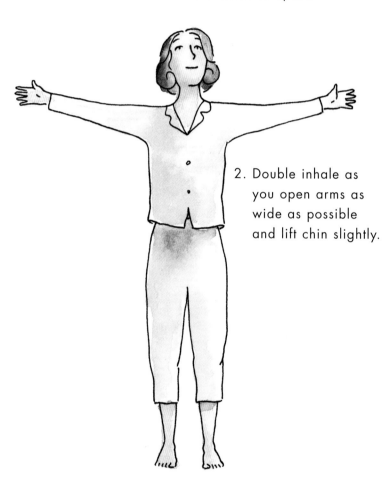

2. Double inhale as you open arms as wide as possible and lift chin slightly.

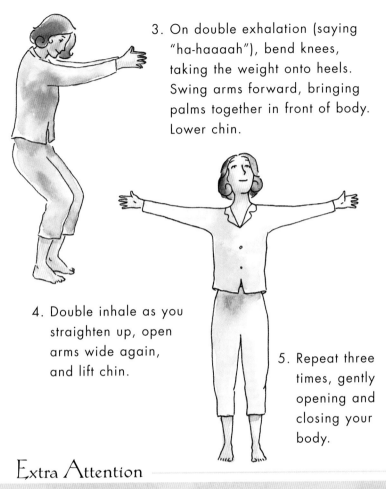

3. On double exhalation (saying "ha-haaaah"), bend knees, taking the weight onto heels. Swing arms forward, bringing palms together in front of body. Lower chin.

4. Double inhale as you straighten up, open arms wide again, and lift chin.

5. Repeat three times, gently opening and closing your body.

Extra Attention

You may occasionally slow this down in order to explore the stretches, but as a warm-up it is done briskly. As you open arms wide, you feel a stretch in the wrists, the forearms and upper arms, even the front of the shoulders. Feel how the heart opens and the spirit lifts. When you swing the arms forward, there's a nice stretch across the upper back and shoulders. Notice if any tension is being held in the jaw or eyes.

Warm-up 2

Breath: double breathing

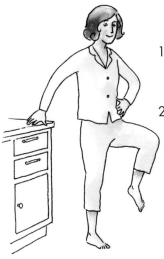

1. Stand near surface to rest hand for balance, if necessary.

2. Double inhale as you raise bent knee.

3. As you double exhale, relax foot and lower without touching floor, then swing straightened leg up with foot flexed. Relax again. Do three times; then rotate ankle three times in each direction. Repeat with other leg.

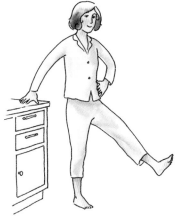

Note

These exercises were taught by Paramahansa Yogananda, an Indian mystic who brought yoga to America in 1920 and established the Self Realization Fellowship. They are the opening to his Energization Series.

Climbing to Heaven

Breath: *ujjayi*

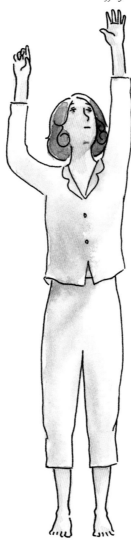

Reach arms high overhead and look up as you "climb," hand over hand, the imaginary rungs of a ladder. This warms the body for the next stretches.

Do seven to ten reaches.

Opening the Heart

Breath: double breathing

1. Inhale. Reach up, bringing palms together. Look up.

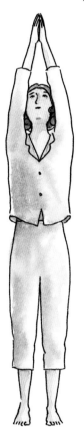

2. Exhale as you bring hands down to prayer position.

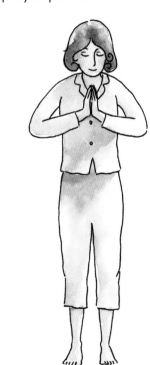

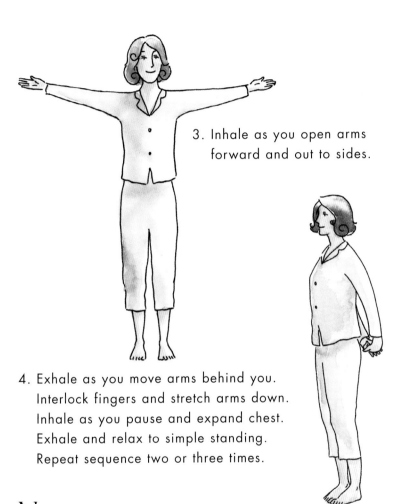

3. Inhale as you open arms forward and out to sides.

4. Exhale as you move arms behind you. Interlock fingers and stretch arms down. Inhale as you pause and expand chest. Exhale and relax to simple standing. Repeat sequence two or three times.

Note

You are already awake now, aren't you? You may feel the energy beginning to flow. If you have a deck, patio, porch, or balcony, try doing these poses out in the open air.

Side Stretch

Breath: *ujjayi*

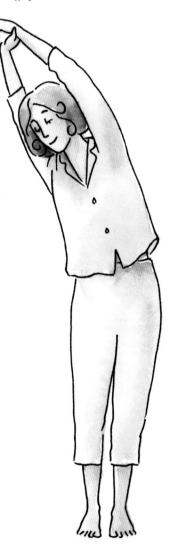

1. Inhale, sweep arms to sides, then overhead. Grasp left wrist.

2. Exhale and bend to right, gently tugging on wrist to stretch left side of body. Look down to keep neck soft. Hold for two or three breaths. Don't force. Stretch just shy of your limits.

3. On an inhalation, return to vertical. Repeat on other side.

Alternate version:

For a more intense stretch, stand sideways to a surface and a few feet away with hand on surface. Arm will be straight to begin. Take other hand high overhead and reach so that body curves. You will feel a wonderful stretch in ribs, skin, and maybe even deep in the abdominal area. As you slightly bend your supporting arm, the stretch increases. Keep both feet firmly planted.
Repeat on other side.

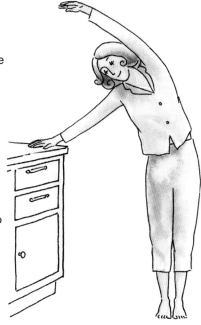

Extra Attention

This is a variation of the half-moon pose. Feel the inbreath expand the ribs and back. If you notice a tendency for the highest shoulder to tilt forward, bring it gently back so that you bend sideways as if between two plates of glass. It is likely that one side is more flexible than the other.

Tree Pose 1

Breath: *ujjayi*

Place sole of one foot on opposite inner thigh. Place it on ankle or calf if it is difficult to reach upper thigh. Toes point down.

Hold for three to five breaths and repeat with other leg.

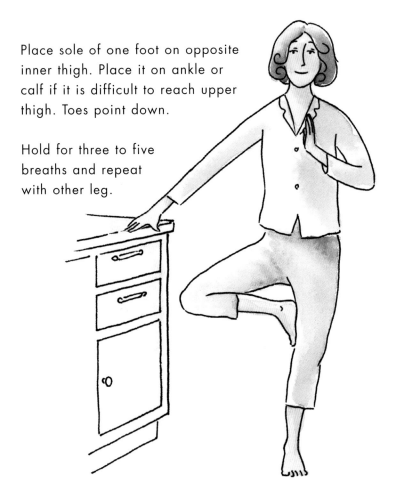

Extra Attention

If you don't need to touch the counter for balance, bring your palms together in prayer position, thumbs touching your heart center. Press palms firmly together to add steadiness to the pose. Pay attention to hugging the standing leg toward the median line of the body and keep growing taller, like a tree. Take the arms overhead, palms facing or touching. Tilt the tailbone down a tiny bit and firm the muscles of the lower abdomen.

Balance is easier if you find a focus point and keep the eyes steady. The breath is moving at all times, deeply and smoothly. Using the *ujjayi* breath and listening to it will help keep you from gripping or holding your breath.

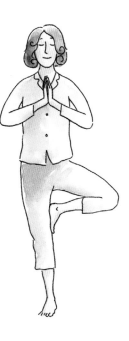

Tree Pose 2 (optional)

Breath: *ujjayi*

This version of the tree pose is more difficult and not suitable for everyone. If you can do it, try alternating it with Tree Pose 1.

Use hands to place foot on front of opposite thigh as near groin as possible with sole facing up. Bent knee is lowered to point down. If foot won't stay up on its own, continue holding it.

Hold for three to five breaths.

Repeat with other leg.

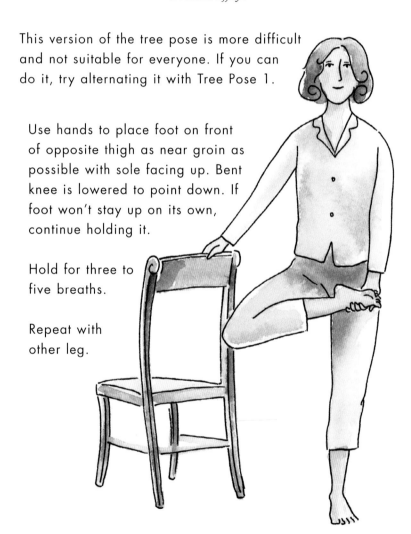

Extra Attention

If this pose causes knee pain use Tree Pose 1. When your balance allows, hold the foot with one hand (if you're holding right foot, use left hand) and reach the other behind the body and grasp your upper arm. Eventually the foot may stay and you can take your hands into prayer position at the heart center.

In standing balance poses, you will strengthen the foot and ankle of the standing leg as well as improve balance. As you become steadier, try closing your eyes. This may strengthen your concentration as you also strengthen your muscles.

Pause for Reflection

Being "in" one of these balance poses, or in any posture, is no different from the way you are "in" any moment of your life. What are the mind's habits? Are you looking ahead to when you have finished this pose and you can go on to the next one? (Just as you look forward to the next situation, the next house, the next relationship, the next week?) How much of our lives are wasted in this way, never fully experiencing where we are at the moment?

Try being in each pose with curiosity. In tree pose, for example, notice the standing foot. As you press the ball of the big toe firmly into the floor, can you also lift the inner arch of the foot? Are your toes relaxed and lengthened, or white from gripping? Is the weight spread evenly on the four corners of the foot? Feel the movement in your ankle as your body tries to maintain balance, compensating first right, then left. Balance in life is just such a series of constant corrections.

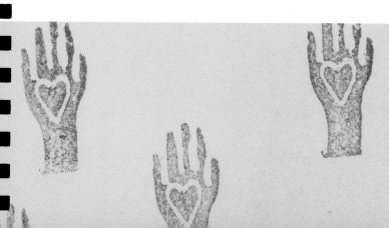

Notice the bent knee; if it is angling forward, can you gently nudge it back and encourage the kneecap to reach down? Check your shoulder blades. Can you broaden and slide them down your back? This helps you to open and lift the chest, but does it increase the arch in the lower back? Can you move the tailbone down slightly as you lengthen the neck? Notice smaller areas, such as the tongue. Is it soft or tense? The jaw and throat? What about the eyes? As you look out, can they be soft and receptive instead of hardened?

The big challenge is to keep the breath flowing smoothly. Focusing on your breath will help quiet the endless commenting of your mind, so you truly can be quietly and fully in the moment. Some days, take tree pose and hold it longer—thirty seconds to a minute, looking intently inward and making your own discoveries. You can take this curiosity into every part of the Morning Cup routine.

Arm Stretches

Breath: *ujjayi*

Drop one hand between shoulder blades, palm facing skin. With other hand, gently press or pull elbow back and toward middle of body. Hold for a breath or two. Repeat on other side.

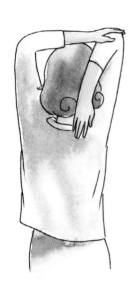

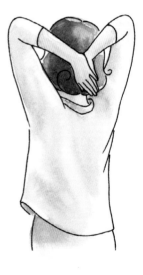

Optional Arm Stretch:

Drop both hands between shoulder blades with palms touching. Bend and straighten arms, keeping elbows hugged close to head. Your hands may not easily reach between the shoulder blades at first. Move in that direction and you will get the stretch. Don't force.

Extra Attention

This is a simple movement but tricky. Observe the neck. Be sensitive and attentive. You will feel a stretch in the upper arms. What else do you feel?

Cactus

Breath: silent or *ujjayi*

1. Back up to a wall with feet as close to wall as possible and head resting on wall.

2. Lift arms, bend elbows, and point fingers up. Fingertips will be in line with ears. Backs of hands are on wall if possible. Don't force. Press small of back toward wall (it doesn't touch) and keep chin level or slightly down. Hold for a few breaths.

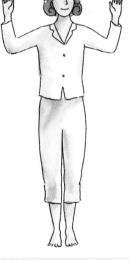

Extra Attention

If your shoulders and arms are tight, or if your upper back has rounded, it may be a challenge to touch the wall with the head, elbows, and hands at the same time. Work gently to roll the shoulders back, and move the shoulder blades deeper into the body. Tilting the pelvis to move the small of the back to the wall adds another challenge. This simple action, practiced daily, may help prevent or correct rounding of the shoulders and upper spine, known as kyphosis. If you are an older person, this is wonderful taken in small amounts daily. Let your mantras be "Breathe" and "Don't strain." You may be using muscles you have neglected. If you feel a strain, do a little less for a few days.

Elbow Circles

Breath: silent or *ujjayi*

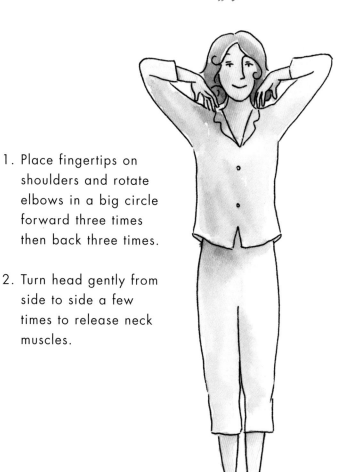

1. Place fingertips on shoulders and rotate elbows in a big circle forward three times then back three times.

2. Turn head gently from side to side a few times to release neck muscles.

Hands

You will sit in a straight chair for the next section. First take a few moments to stretch your hands.

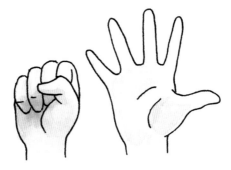

1. Alternately make a fist and stretch hands wide.

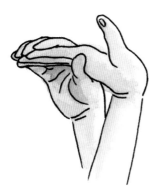

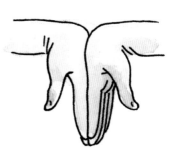

2. Pull your fingers back.   3. Counter-stretch wrists.

Arch and Curl

Breath: *ujjayi*

1. Sit on front edge of chair, feet flat on floor under knees. Place hands on thighs near knees. Inhale, arch back, puff out chest, and lift chin until you feel your throat stretch.

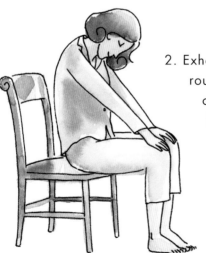

2. Exhale and hollow belly as you round forward, dropping chin on chest. This is a continuous flowing movement. Repeat several times, pausing for a few seconds in your extreme positions.

Hip Stretch

Breath: silent

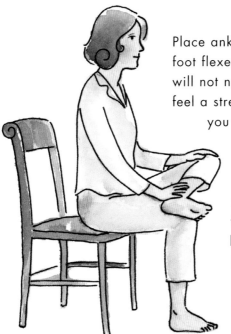

Place ankle on opposite leg with foot flexed. Sit tall. Most people will not need to lean forward to feel a stretch in the hip area. If you are very flexible in the hips, you may want to fold forward a little, but stay in your comfort zone. You don't want to feel any strain in the knee, so keep the foot firmly flexed. Hold for three to five breaths. Repeat on other side.

Extra Attention

Observe the amount of curve in your lower back; the slightest change there affects the stretch. Notice the height of the bent leg's knee. Is one side more lifted? Wait in this position for five or six breaths. As you breathe in, imagine that the inhaled breath goes all the way to your tailbone. As you exhale, imagine that the breath lengthens the spine, causing you to get taller. Think of those curled paper party favors that straighten out as you blow through them.

Pause for Reflection

As you hold any pose, breathing, you may notice the beginnings of impatience. Just observe that feeling, but don't act on it. We all tend to want something to be going on every minute. We have the habit of jumping up and running away from discomfort or boredom, as well as from pain and sorrow. In yoga you get to practice the pause. Learn to be comfortable with stillness. Then, out in the world, when you must wait, as in airports, doctors' offices, and in traffic, you may learn to look at these times as little islands of rest in an otherwise turbulent river. Even if you don't always welcome them, you can remain peaceful and accept them when they come.

Knee Squeeze

Breath: silent

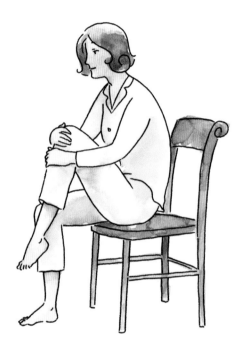

Use both hands to pull knee toward chest. As you lift your foot from floor use your abdominal muscles by pulling them toward the spine rather than letting them bulge and thicken. Keep them active throughout the lift. Hold knee for a few moments then lower it back to the floor. Do each leg two times.

Twists

1. Sit tall with feet together and shins vertical.

2. Slowly twist body to left and look over shoulder. Don't push past your comfortable limit.

3. Reach right arm across knees to outside of left thigh and apply gentle leverage. Don't force neck. Think of your chin as floating in the direction of your shoulder.

4. Stay for three deep breaths; then unwind to front. Repeat on other side.

Optional Neck Stretches:

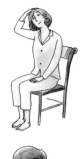

1. Drop ear toward right shoulder. Reach right arm across top of head. Gently rest right hand on head with fingers near left ear. Stay a few breaths, then repeat on other side.

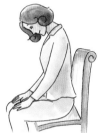

2. Drop chin and lift chest up to meet it to lengthen back of neck. Stay a few breaths.

Extra Attention

Be aware of any discomfort in the lower back or neck. Always stay within your comfort zone. Think about distributing the twist equally along the spine so that the twist is not concentrated in the area of one overly flexible section. Pay attention to each vertebra, asking each to turn a little. Keep the spine lengthening up and hips firmly grounded. As an option, continue turning the head back and forth as you maintain the twist. This action stimulates the throat.

Twists improve the health of the discs and keep the spine resilient. They gently compress your organs and can have a detoxifying effect on the system. If you do these twists every day, you will always be able to back your car out of your driveway.

Tiptoe Strengthener

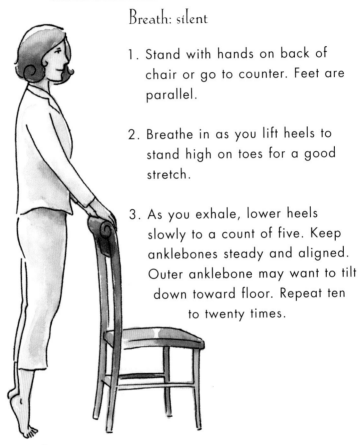

Breath: silent

1. Stand with hands on back of chair or go to counter. Feet are parallel.

2. Breathe in as you lift heels to stand high on toes for a good stretch.

3. As you exhale, lower heels slowly to a count of five. Keep anklebones steady and aligned. Outer anklebone may want to tilt down toward floor. Repeat ten to twenty times.

Extra Attention

This is strengthening for the feet and calf muscles. The challenge is to not let the feet wobble as the heels come down. The slower you lower, the more strengthening it will be. What part of the heel do you land on? Keep an eye on the inner anklebones and make sure you keep them steady.

Hamstring Strengtheners

Breath: *ujjayi*

1. Face a surface for support. Hips are squared to front as you lift your straightened leg behind, toe pointed. Toe may be only a few inches from floor. Stand tall as you lift and lower leg. Do a series of three lifts, barely touching floor with toe when you lower leg. On third lift, hold for a few seconds. Do sequence twice with each leg.

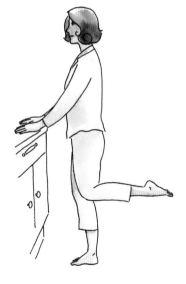

2. Fold and unfold knee, squeezing heel toward buttocks. Keep knees in line with each other if you can. Do two times with each leg.

Hamstring Strengtheners (continued)

Breath: *ujjayi*

3. Combine 1 & 2 from previous page. Lift leg straight behind; lower to starting position, then bend knee and stretch foot toward buttock. Do three times with each leg.

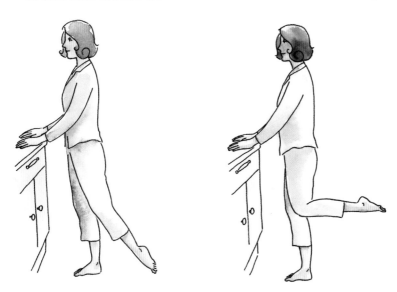

Extra Attention

Squeeze rather than kick when you make these movements. Is one side stronger than the other? Most bodies have a dominant side. Sometimes one hamstring is stronger than the other. Maybe you can feel some of the other muscles that help to lift and fold the leg. This strengthens and tones them all.

Stork (optional)

Breath: *ujjayi*

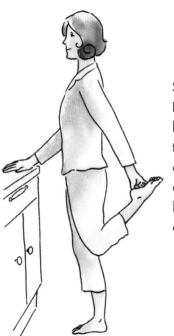

Stand balanced on one foot. Fold other leg behind and hold foot. Use free hand to touch something for balance, or take it straight up overhead. Hold for several breaths and repeat with other leg.

Extra Attention

Try to keep the knees in line with each other, but don't force it. You will feel a stretch in the thigh. As the quadricep muscles begin to lengthen with this practice, lining up the knees will become easier. Don't overstretch the knee. There is a tendency for the lower back to overarch. Counteract by lengthening the tailbone down.

Push-ups

Breath: *ujjayi*

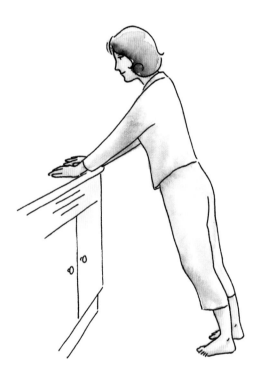

1. Step both feet back from counter, sink, or stove.
   Place hands on front edge, shoulder width apart.

2. With elbows hugged close and body straight, bend
   arms and lower chest toward counter. Lift chin slightly
   and firm the abdominal muscles. Stay broad between
   the shoulder blades. Push back by straightening your
   arms. Heels may not stay on floor, but stretch them in
   that direction. Don't let shoulders hunch toward ears.

   Repeat up to ten times.

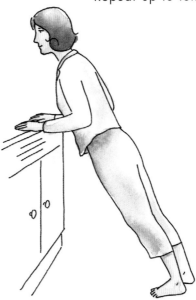

Extra Attention

This is a modification of the classic push-up. If you have no
upper body strength and this is hard for you, begin with just a
few. Ask yourself, "What part of this can I do?" If you can only
lean forward a tiny bit and hold for a few breaths, do it. If one
is a challenge, then just do one. To maximize the strengthening
benefit, pause at the halfway point and go even slower .

Warrior 1

Breath: *ujjayi*

1. Face counter with toes of one foot near cabinet. Stretch other leg back two to three feet as you bend front knee keeping shin vertical. Bring toes of back foot to point toward counter, but keep foot firmly on floor.

2. Although thigh of back leg is turned out, try to turn front of body to face counter without twisting back knee. Place hands on counter and gently exert a downward pressure, to lift chest and collarbones. Move shoulder blades down the back.

3. After a few breaths, lift chin and look up a bit, feeling a stretch in your throat, but don't crunch the back of your neck, particularly if you have neck problems. Repeat on other side.

Extra Attention

Experiment with the distance between your feet. You want to feel an arching of the upper back without a crunch in the lower back. To prevent taking too much of the arch into the lower back, provide a resistance by slightly tucking the tailbone down. Lift the chest and tuck the tailbone, back and forth, splitting the difference. This is what Rodney Yee calls "creating a dialogue."

If you support the knee against the cabinet, the knee may extend forward past vertical a little. If you have knee problems or feel this stresses the knee, keep the knee directly over the ankle.

After holding this position for some time, and if your balance will allow, lift your arms overhead, palms either touching or facing each other, and look up. Keeping your weight strongly in both feet will help with balance. Don't forget to keep the breath flowing smoothly and deeply!

Caution

If you are an older person or suspect that you may have heart trouble, don't lift the arms overhead.

Flat Back Stretch

Breath: silent

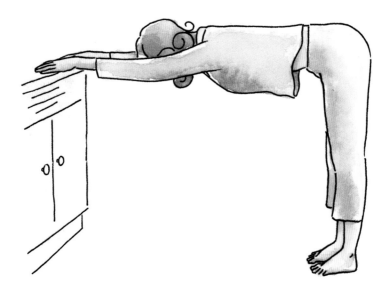

With hands on counter, step away until back is flat. Arms and legs are straight, and hips are over ankles. If back is rounded because hamstrings are tight, bend knees a little. Lengthen whole back including back of neck. Stay for a few moments breathing up and down spine.

This is a stretch for arms, too, and a neutralizing pose after the backbending of Warrior 1.

Warrior 3 (optional)

Breath: *ujjayi*

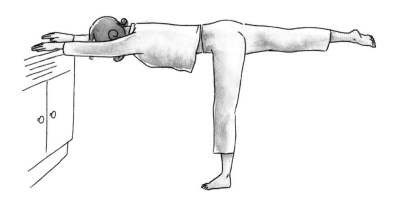

From flat back stretch bring feet together. Lift one leg behind as high as you can but no higher than parallel to floor. This is a supported version of Warrior 3 and is very strengthening for the standing leg. Hands are offering support, but you can play with balancing. Hold as long as you like and enjoy. Picture yourself as an ice skater! Repeat with other leg. (If you are wondering about Warrior 2, it is a more advanced pose not appropriate to the scope of this routine.)

Leg Stretch

Breath: silent or *ujjayi*

Be careful getting into and out
of this pose. Situate yourself
near a chair and a stable
surface that you can put one
or both hands on.

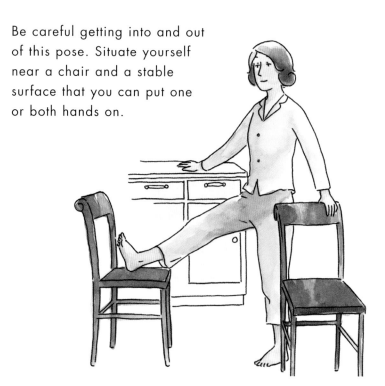

1. Stabilize yourself using chairback and countertop. Face
   second chair seat with feet parallel on floor. Place one
   heel on chair seat and flex foot. If this is no stretch,
   add a cookbook or phone book under foot for extra
   height. If still no stretch, try placing heel higher, using
   more books. Hold for three to five breaths.

2. With foot still on chair and one or both hands on other chair for support, turn body sidewise, away from lifted foot by pivoting standing foot 90 degrees. Feel a stretch in inner thigh. Hold for three to five breaths. Pay attention to rotating the thigh of your lifted leg outwards (backwards) while keeping knee and toes pointing toward ceiling. Be cautious as you come out of this pose. Pivot standing foot to face chair again, and hold on to a surface before you lift foot down from chair seat. Repeat with other leg.

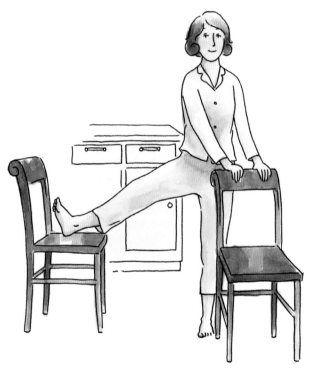

Leg Stretch (continued)

Breath: silent or *ujjayi*

Extra Attention

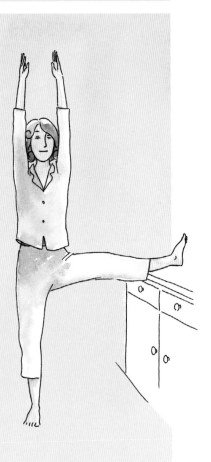

With daily practice you will notice improved flexibility very quickly. Work to keep the pelvis fairly even. Slightly hollow the belly, and avoid letting the lower back arch too much. Don't get ambitious and risk overstretching the hamstrings. Always work in a gentle way and remember to breathe, paying attention to the tight places. If your balance is excellent, you may reach your arms straight overhead, lifting your torso up and away from the hips, but remember to hold on to a surface as you transition out of this pose.

Forward Bend

Breath: silent

This standing forward bend is not recommended for persons with back problems or glaucoma. If in doubt about this or the modified version (crossed arms on countertop), please consult your healthcare provider.

Rest hands or head (whichever is more comfortable) on chair seat. Back will be rounded and knees slightly bent. Stay as long as you like. Bend knees and slowly roll up to standing. If you feel a momentary dizziness, pause and let the blood pressure come back to normal. Do one time.

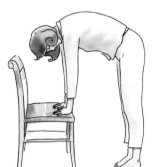

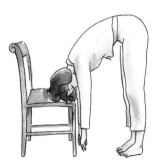

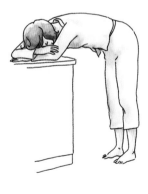

Hungry Lion

Breath: *ujjayi*

Take a deep breath. As you exhale, stretch arms straight forward with fingers spread. Open eyes wide, stick out tongue, and try to touch tongue to chin. Hold with breath out a few seconds, experiencing the tension in throat and face, then release. Repeat.

Extra Attention

Hungry Lion brings extra blood to the throat area and is a very good practice to ward off a sore throat. When you feel the first warning tickle of a sore throat, do this throughout the day as you think of it. It has worked for me many times.

Mountain Pose

Breath: silent

And so you end the routine
with Mountain Pose, the
basic standing meditative
pose. Stand with feet
together or a few inches
apart, upper body lifted
off hips, back of the
neck long, hands
relaxed at your sides.
Close your eyes.

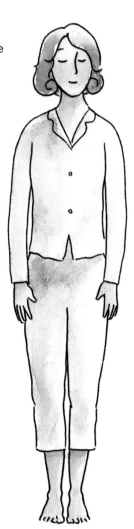

Mountain Pose (continued)

Breath: silent

Extra Attention

Be aware of your feet connecting you to earth. Feel the weight of your body falling on to the front of the heels. Consciously relax the eyes, jaw, and throat. Soften everything without sagging. Allow the breath to become deeper and more silent. With each outbreath let tension drain from your arms and legs. You may feel the subtle and continuous effort within your body to orient itself in space and maintain balance. Notice both feet, letting each carry an equal part of your weight.

Stand quietly, appreciating the gentle, natural flowing rhythm of your breath and what your body could do today. When at last you open your eyes, let them be soft and settled back into the skull, so that you look out at the world from a deep place within. Open your ears and allow hearing, noting the various sounds that arise and pass away. Experience the world directly.

You may occasionally experience brief moments of absolute stillness and peace, feeling yourself at home in your body and at home with your breath, in the safe harbor of your deepest self.

Standing Meditation

As you stand in Mountain Pose at the end of your Morning Cup, take a moment to form an intention for the day. Intentions have great power. We all get off track and lose the path we want to be on. If we keep coming back to our intention, eventually the road will go that way. Here are some sample intentions, but you will know what your heart yearns for.

>Today I will practice generosity.
>I will be more patient with ....
>I will notice my feelings and try to feel my feelings instead of shoving them under.
>I will listen to other points of view, without trying to push my own agenda.
>I will respond lovingly when others are upset.
>I will remember to stop at moments throughout the day, breathe deeply, and relax every part of my body.
>Today I will focus on the blessings in my life.

Now you are through. Whether or not you get to your mat or a class today, you can be satisfied that you have covered your bases. Your body has gotten its daily cleansing and tune-up. Let this program become as much a part of your day as brushing your teeth. Try it every day for two or three weeks and observe the changes you are experiencing.

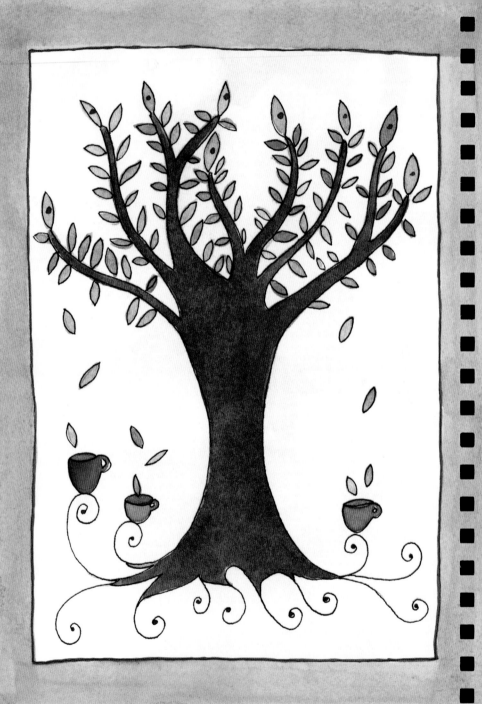

If You'd Like to Learn More

A Morning Cup of Yoga is not meant to take the place of a longer practice, but don't underestimate the power of this modest, daily routine. Once you have begun to benefit from the Morning Cup routine, I hope you will be inspired to learn more about this life-changing system. The following section is intended to answer some of the questions you may have about yoga and help you understand more about its physical and spiritual benefits.

Bringing Mind and Body Together

Some people take the word yoga to mean the training of the body through yoga postures. But yoga is more than just exercise—it's a complete system for living harmoniously in the world and for attaining peace. In Sanskrit, *yoga* can be understood at different levels. For instance, yoga, meaning yoke or union, can be interpreted to mean the unifying of body, breath, and mind.

Gyms and health clubs borrow heavily these days from the yoga tradition, but an important difference between doing exercises and practicing yoga is the level of attention and awareness you bring to the work. In yoga you are developing a relationship to the breath with the intention of bringing body, breath, and mind into one single awareness in the present moment.

With yoga we learn to work with the body using concentrated attention. Yoga poses, or *asanas*, are mostly done slowly with constant observation. An advanced practitioner of yoga is not the one who can do the most amazing feats of strength or balance, but the one who can pay closer attention and modulate his effort and breath appropriately.

Improving Your Posture

One of the results of practicing the yoga *asanas* is the improvement of your posture. Your mother was right. It's important to stand up straight! How we hold our bodies has an influence on our mind and emotions. Try slumping in an exaggerated way and right away you feel defeated, dull, discouraged. Slump in only a slight way, and still there is a sense of low energy, a laxness. On the other hand, stand tall, with heart center open and lifted, legs strong and resolute, and feet firmly planted on the earth. There is an instant translation to the psyche. Don't you feel the difference? You feel stronger and more empowered.

Sometimes poor posture is just a bad habit we acquire along the way. But often a collapsed posture originates in your feeling about yourself. You are not alone if you experience feelings of powerlessness or shame. The idea that we are not okay—not enough—seems to be built into our culture. For many, trying to conform to or overcome a constraining self-image is a source of constant frustration.

Unblocking Your Energy Flow

As you begin to use yoga to rid your body of unnecessary tension, you will have more energy—energy that you can use in something far more fun and productive than gripping your jaw, hunching your shoulders, and clenching your teeth or belly. I'm sure you have noticed that energy mysteriously comes and goes. At intervals you may feel bogged down and lackluster for no apparent reason. Something is blocking the flow of your energy. Those times can be a clue that something is going on in your mind/body that you need to investigate.

Facing a task you don't want to do or a situation you don't know how to solve is a major thief of vitality. Ask yourself, "What am I resisting here?" Being conflicted about something can paralyze you. So look deeper. Ask yourself, "What is the outcome I really want here?" When you become clearer and know the path you want, your energy will come back.

As you begin the practice of yoga, you will start to notice the mind/body relationship. When you feel tensions in the body, you will have the choice and the ability to release them. When anxiety nibbles at you, you can ask, "Where is that anxiety registered in the body?" Just a fleeting thought or image across the sky of your mind can cause something in your body to clench and contract. But if you are not looking, you may miss those connections. When you follow the body's clues and discover emotion that may have been hidden, you have taken a first step toward freedom.

Other blocks to a free flow of energy—besides chronic tension, poor posture, and negative thinking—are eating devitalized food, and loss of contact with fresh air and sunlight. We humans were meant to live and walk on the earth, not be confined to buildings and artificial light. So get out in nature as much as possible. Go barefoot. Reconnect with the vitality and energy of the earth.

A Sip of Sutras

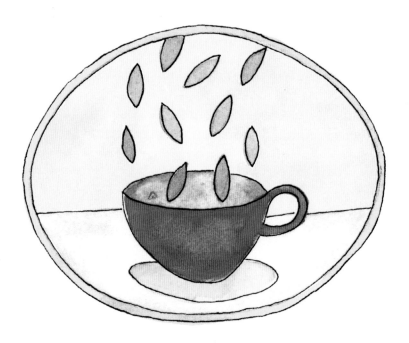

The physical part of yoga is important, but what good is a strong resilient body if your heart is closed, and your mind is imprisoned by your ego and its demands? What good is an attractive appearance if you are deceitful or unkind? What good is physical health if you are miserable because you have what you don't want, and don't have what you do want? What good is energy and vitality if it is used to cause harm?

At their deepest level, the physical practices of yoga exist within a spiritual framework whose ultimate goal is the union (*yoga*) of the individual soul with the divine—a melting of the individual personality into pure consciousness. The physical postures are seen as a preparation for spiritual liberation.

The path to this spiritual liberation is outlined in the Sutras of Patanjali, an ancient codification of the system of yoga. The eight steps of the classical yoga system recorded in this Sanskrit work are composed of the *yamas* and *niyamas* (ethical precepts), *asanas* (ease and steadiness in the body), *pranayama* (breath and energy control), and the stages of meditation. It is beyond the scope of this little book to do more than take a small sip of this system, but let's have a brief look at the ethical precepts and the practice of meditation.

Yamas and Niyamas

The first two steps of the system of yoga, the *yamas* and *niyamas*, are foundational for anyone embarking on a serious yoga path. These ethical precepts are guidelines designed to help a human being live a wholesome life in harmony with self and others. The five *yamas*, or restraints, focus on your relationships to the outer world. The five *niyamas*, or observances, are personal cleansing and self-training practices.

An interesting and productive practice is to choose one and keep it as a focus for a day, a week, or more, and monitor your relationship to it. Put a list of precepts next to your Morning Cup outline, and think about them often. As you work with these precepts, you will find they twine in and out, connecting with each other.

Yamas

Non-violence (*Ahimsa*)

In the first precept, we investigate what constitutes violence. Thich Nhat Hanh, a Vietnamese monk who dedicated his life to teaching people how to create peace, says that when we are irritated, already that is violence in "seed" form. When we are upset with someone, when a critical thought arises, this is violence. When we speak with harshness or in the veiled form of implied criticism, this is violence because there is the intention to harm.

Perhaps we are basically violent toward ourselves. We criticize ourselves without mercy. Look deeply and you will start to notice when violence arises in you. Where is it coming from? What hidden angers or fears are simmering there? A frustration in the outer world can open a channel to those angers and fears that can erupt as aggression.

Just seeing and truthfully acknowledging our own violent impulses begins to reveal what is fueling those impulses. With understanding, gentleness and compassion can unfold. True harmlessness begins with ourselves.

Truthfulness (*Satya*)

To tell the truth, most of us don't tell the truth! To work with this precept, just watch all the ways you devise to bend the truth a little bit. Doesn't putting on makeup qualify as a little lie? We lie for many reasons: to spare someone's feelings, to protect ourselves or our reputations, to avoid confrontation. When you choose this precept to work on, you can investigate your reasons for not telling the truth.

Is it possible to live without lying, without subterfuge? This precept is worth thinking about, and experimenting with. Telling the truth can be a freeing experience, but we must be careful that we don't use truth as an excuse to injure. To tell the truth, and give no harm—that is the challenge. To adhere to truthfulness takes a strong clear attention.

Non-stealing or Non-coveting (*Asteya*)

To covet what another has comes from a sense of lack. To steal is to take anything that has not been offered freely. This might include the casual taking of a flower from a neighbor's yard, or a grape at the grocery store. How many temptations there are daily! On a larger scale, stealing can also be interpreted to mean taking more than you need, thus depriving others. Consumer cultures such as ours are stealing the earth's resources. When we use more than we need of electricity, fuels, water, we are stealing. When we poison the earth, our rivers and air, we are stealing from all the beings who share the planet with us.

The sutras promise that the perfection of each *yama* and *niyama* brings with it a reward. To be steady in *asteya* is to always have all that is needed. If we all took only what we needed, and respected the needs of other beings, what a different world this could be.

Chastity (*Brahmacharya*)

Much controversy surrounds the precept *brahmacharya*. Some yoga writings suggest that *brahmacharya* means not celibacy but appropriate sexual behavior. Others define it as moderation in all things (see *The Heart of Yoga* by T.K.V. Desikachar). Some translators say the real meaning of *brahmacharya* is to walk close to God and to be godlike in all of our actions.

There's no doubt that sexuality holds a distorted and inflated status in our culture. Sexuality as pursued by humans is often reduced to a recreation, a contact sport, a diversion, and a tool of the ego. So what does this precept ask us to do with sexual energy?

Energy is just energy. It can take various forms and be channeled according to one's wishes. It is quite possible to use one's vitality for pursuits other than satisfying sexual desire. To take a serious look at this *yama* might be to reassess the priority we have given to sexuality.

🍃 Greedlessness (*Aparigraha*)

Why do we accumulate so much stuff? One reason is the pleasure we get when we buy something we've desired. Second, shopping and acquiring a lot of material possessions may be an attempt to fill an inner emptiness and distract us from the lack of meaning in our lives. Third, we give ourselves status through the amount and quality of our possessions.

For some of us, hoarding is due to a lack of trust that we will have what we need at some future date. Anyone who has lived during a difficult time of want or privation and suffered a real lack (such as during the Depression) is especially prone to hoarding.

Accumulating an excess of material goods does not make our lives meaningful. Duane Elgin in his persuasive book *Voluntary Simplicity* writes, "We need little when we are directly in touch with life. It is when we remove ourselves from direct and wholehearted participation in life that emptiness and boredom creep in."

Niyamas

🍃 Purity (*Saucha*)

Saucha refers to purification of mind and body. The yoga postures and breathing are purifying practices that help the body get rid of impurities, but we also must pay close attention to what we eat and drink. Whatever is taken into the body will affect the mind/body.

Unfortunately, much of our food is grown in depleted soil and is subjected to pesticides and other chemicals. Some foods are being altered at the genetic level, and no one yet knows the effect this will have. Foods are grown far away from market and have lost freshness and food value by the time they reach us. So, the situation is not ideal. Still, we can try to find organic food grown close to home. And we can be as mindful as possible about what we put into our bodies.

To purify the mind and psyche is another aspect of *saucha*. The discipline of a daily meditation practice is deeply cleansing. Just sitting in stillness and observing whatever arises is indispensable for growth. I have also found that intensive meditation retreats have a powerful cleansing effect.

Practice of contentment (*Santosa*)

A beautiful *niyama* to work with is the practice of contentment, or *santosa*. In this practice, we decide that in this very moment we will be contented, no matter what storms are threatening. The fact is, there are always storms. If we wait for things to become as we demand them to be in order to be contented, we will always be waiting. Contentment can be enjoyed in small tastes. On the worst of days, it's possible to pause and look at the world with unclouded eyes for a moment, see the sky, hear a bird, see a child's face and say, "For this tiny moment I choose to be contented."

Begin to look for those moments. When you crawl into your bed at night, let your body relax. Let go of the concerns of your day. Stop trying to control events and people around you, and, as the Beatles said, "Let It Be." When we quit fighting and resisting, contentment arises naturally.

Right effort (*Tapas*)

This *niyama* refers to self-discipline and/or ascetic practices that develop willpower. In simple terms, *tapas* involves making the effort and commitment to do something that is difficult. To make progress in any pursuit requires *tapas*. The musician must practice and practice, willing himself through the low ebb times of resistance or boredom. The athlete hones his skills with years of dedicated effort.

Going for the gold in any arena means learning to ignore the voice that says, "This isn't comfortable. This isn't fun." Staying with any difficult task creates an inner strength. The fire of the effort purifies and tempers the will as the furnace tempers steel to create a fine sword. But, remember, yoga is about balance. Effort must somehow be coupled with steadiness and ease, so that one is never lost inside a consuming fire. The two wings of yoga, both of which must work, are effort and surrender. Perhaps the steadiness and ease come from truly accepting the outcome—whatever it may be.

Self-study (Svadhyaya)

Sva means "self" and adhyaya means "inquiry" or "examination." This niyama can be summed up as "Know Thyself." Self-observation, a willingness to uncover and dismantle one's delusions—this is hard work! We develop a self-image, a complex system of values, a concept of the world, certain patterns of behavior and strategies. In short we create a movie, cast ourselves as the star, get on stage, and spend the rest of our life acting out the script.

We invent ourselves and then we are imprisoned by our invention. We think we are in control of our life, that we are making our own choices, when in reality the choices are being made for us by our movie script. This is a form of bondage. In yoga, the veil that covers the reality of who we really are is called avidya, which means self-ignorance. The system of yoga will begin to thin this veil.

In addition to yoga and meditation, many people find occasional therapy to be useful. A discerning therapist can help us see and address our blind spots. So often our reactions to people and events are automatic responses that come from below the level of consciousness. Seeing our patterns gives us the opportunity to make choices.

We can see a lot even without help if we decide to get quiet, start looking, and be fearless with our inquiry. Keeping a journal has been a major clarifier for me, as has meditation.

✍ Surrender to God *(Isvara pranidhana)*

This *niyama* has been translated variously as devotion to God, yielding of all actions to God, contemplation of God, or surrender to God. *Isvara* is one of the many Sanskrit names for God. All religions, large or tribal, have a name for the Supreme Being. Yoga is not a religion, but it does acknowledge the indivisible mystery. The practices of yoga are not at odds with any religion and can actually enrich one's relationship to one's religion.

However we envision or name God, we realize the human mind cannot possibly grasp the full picture and that even our vision of God is limited because we are limited. We are part of a great reality that is too big for us to see or understand. Everything is intricately interrelated. Whatever is done or said reverberates throughout the cosmos. It is said that the beat of a butterfly's wings affects the world's climate. All we can do is act on our best information, with the best knowledge we have, and with the kindest motives, and then leave the results to God.

There are many translations of the sutras and there seem to be many different views on the precepts, and how to work with them. You can find those who view the *yamas* and *niyamas* as models of behavior, something to be aspired to. There are others who say that they are the states that naturally arise in us, like fruits borne on a tree, when we realize the truth of who we really are and the interconnectedness of all things.

Meditation

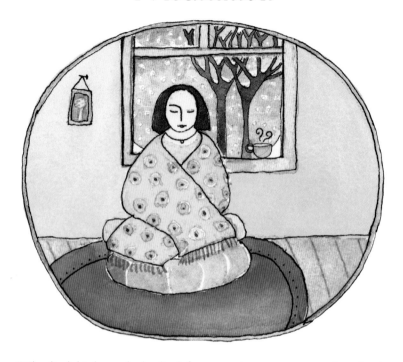

"What lies behind us and what lies before us are tiny matters compared to what lies within us." —Ralph Waldo Emerson

We are living in the noisiest and busiest culture ever. There's hardly a moment when we are not bombarded with stimulation. Meditation can be an island of peace in the midst of that and it can also have a clarifying and calming effect on your life. If you sit quietly for a little while every day, you will be rewarded.

The physical benefits of meditation have been recognized by the medical community. Studies at Harvard, the Menninger Clinic, and the stress reduction clinic at the University of Massachusetts

Medical Center, among others, have shown that meditation significantly lowers blood pressure, decreases pain, improves the immune system by reducing stress, and brings a more positive outlook. In other words, meditation is good for you! If it were a pill, we would all have a bottle in our medicine cabinets.

So what is the reluctance to sitting down and being quiet and having nothing going on? It's unfamiliar! It feels very strange to have nothing "happening." When one sits down for the first time, just sitting still is a great challenge. So, for starters, one should say to oneself, "For this short period I am willing to experience boredom, restlessness, and even discomfort. I will sit here and not let those feelings drive me away from my intent."

Decide that you will sit for a little while every day for at least two weeks. Gradually your body will get used to it. This is an inward expedition, and will become, over time, far from boring. Here are some simple steps to guide you.

Create Your Own Space

Designate a space that has room for a chair or cushion, and maybe a picture that inspires you. Make your place as simple or elaborate as you wish. If you like incense, by all means use it. Create an atmosphere of quiet reflection. I have a bell and a timer and begin and end each session by ringing the bell. With repetition, the mind comes to know that it's time to settle, and will do so quicker. Decide how long you are going to sit. Begin with ten or fifteen minutes. As the weeks go on, you can increase the time to thirty or forty-five minutes a day.

Choose a Time

Try to sit at the same time every day. Early morning is ideal, before the mind gets revved up to its habitual speeds. The energy of the earth is quieter in the mornings and so are you. But any time of the day you can work out is better than no time. Have a big drink of water (always a good idea on rising), shower, or at least splash your face with water. Stretch the body a little if there's time and then sit down.

Learn to Sit

Come to your chair or cushion as if you were coming home and could finally rest. Throw a shawl or sweater around your shoulders for warmth and adjust your spine so that it is upright without force. Try to maintain the natural curves of the spine. Lower your chin slightly to lengthen the back of the neck. Find as comfortable a posture as you can, and then sit still. It takes a while for the body to accustom itself. New muscles are called into play, but they will strengthen over time.

Calm the Mind

Sit down, close the eyes, become still, and allow your attention to shift inward. At first you can observe physical sensations; the rise and fall of the belly and chest, air movement on the skin, sounds as they arise and vibrate in your ears. Go through the body systematically relaxing each part: the face, the shoulders, etc. Become aware of the weight of the body on the cushion or chair seat. You may want to stay in this phase for a while before focusing on the breath alone.

Observe the inhalations and exhalations and notice the way the ribs expand and the belly rises and falls. You can also feel the touch of the breath in the nostrils. There is a pause that occurs when the breath turns—that moment when the exhale has finished but the inhale has not yet begun. In that pause, there is a possible moment of complete stillness. The other turn, usually shorter, occurs when the inhaled breath is "full" and the body lets go into the exhalation.

After a few minutes of these observations, which help you bring your focus inside, you can begin counting the breath. Count down from ten to one, or from one to ten.

Right away you will see that the mind wants to jump to something more interesting. When you notice that you have been thinking and not keeping your focus on the breath, gently bring your attention back to the breath again. Don't be impatient or frustrated. The very act of noticing that you have left the present moment and are out somewhere in never-never land is the practice. You are doing it! Each time you bring the mind back and bid it to "stay," you are strengthening your ability to come into the present moment. That other world, with its images of the past and future, where most of us hang out a lot, is a dream world. It exists only within the imagination.

Observe, Don't Act

An important aspect of a sitting practice is to have no expectations. Now this is truly radical and unfamiliar to us. We are used to reacting—immediately. If we itch, we scratch; if we feel discomfort, we adjust our position. This carries into every area of our lives. Get tired of a job—quit. Get angry—blow up at someone. Have trouble in a relationship—leave it. To break that connection, to see impulses arise and not act on them, but simply to observe them—this is to turn off your auto-pilot. This is the beginning of actually taking control of your life. Simply creating some space between an event and your reaction will have a profound effect on your life.

Find the Quiet

There are many wonderful books and tapes on the subject of meditation by extraordinary teachers. (A few are listed in the Recommended Reading section at the end of this book.) But the main thing is for you to just get started. If you will sit down and be very still for a little while every day, you will reap more rewards than you can imagine.

There is a still voice of wisdom within you. But until you get quiet enough to access it, you may not even know it is there. The thinking mind is similar to a child with a stick stirring a mud puddle. When the busy mind quits churning up the water and allows it to get still, the mud settles to the bottom. The moments when your mind finally becomes quiet and clear, no matter how brief, are a real treasure and the effect can be felt for several hours or all day. A tiny taste of that stillness every day can transform your life.

An Extra Sip

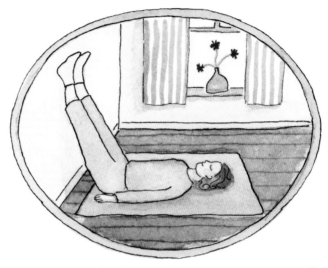

I can't let this little book go without suggesting a taste of a very, very gentle yoga position that has a great restoring effect on your mind/body. It is so simple and yet so powerful. Its yoga name is *Viparita Karani*. But it's called "feet up the wall." And it is just that. When you can catch five minutes for yourself, perhaps at the end of the workday, lie on your back with your hips close to a wall. Swing your legs up, letting the feet rest on the wall. Lengthen the neck by drawing the chin in slightly. Take a few deep breaths and consciously instruct your feet, legs, shoulders, belly, and face to let go and relax.

This mild inversion gives a rest to the heart, lets the venous blood drain from the feet and legs, brings extra nourishment to the brain, clears your thinking, and like the slant board of old, improves your complexion. Perhaps you can find a private place at work, or do it first thing when you come home. This can be practiced any time to drain tension, clear your mind, and refresh your energy.

The Routine at a Glance

After you are familiar with the poses, you can follow this
sequence without reading the complete text. But every now and
then go back and read the instructions again to check up. On
mornings when you have extra time, you can increase repetitions
and extend holding times.

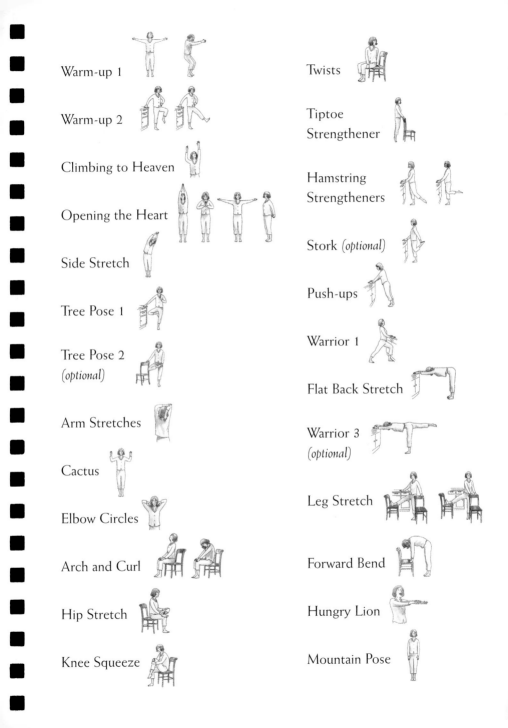

Warm-up 1

Warm-up 2

Climbing to Heaven

Opening the Heart

Side Stretch

Tree Pose 1

Tree Pose 2 *(optional)*

Arm Stretches

Cactus

Elbow Circles

Arch and Curl

Hip Stretch

Knee Squeeze

Twists

Tiptoe Strengthener

Hamstring Strengtheners

Stork *(optional)*

Push-ups

Warrior 1

Flat Back Stretch

Warrior 3 *(optional)*

Leg Stretch

Forward Bend

Hungry Lion

Mountain Pose

Recommended Reading

Beck, Charlotte Joko. *Everyday Zen.* Harper and Row, 1989

Benson, Herbert, M.D. *The Relaxation Response.* HarperCollins, 2000

Desikachar, T.K.V. *The Heart of Yoga.* Inner Traditions International, 1999

Elgin, Duane. *Voluntary Simplicity.* William Morrow and Co., 1981

Hart, William. *Vipassana Meditation as Taught by S. N. Goenka.* HarperCollins, 1987

Iyengar, B.K.S. *Yoga, The Path to Holistic Health.* DK Publishing, 2001

Jensen, Bernard. *Vibrant Health from Your Kitchen.* Bernard Jensen International, 1986

Kabat-Zinn, Jon. *Full Catastrophe Living.* Bantam-Doubleday Dell Publishing Group, 1990

Kornfield, Jack. *A Path with Heart.* Bantam, 1993

Rosen, Richard. *The Yoga of Breath.* Shambhala Press, 2002

Schiffmann, Erich. *Yoga, The Spirit and Practice of Moving Into Stillness.* Pocket Books, 1996

Silva, Mira and Shyam Mehta. *Yoga, The Iyengar Way.* Alfred A. Knopf, 1990

Yee, Rodney. *Yoga, The Poetry of the Body.* Thomas Dunne Books, 2002